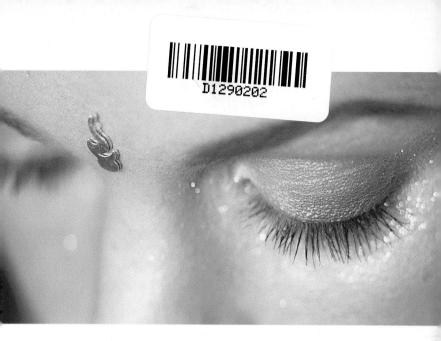

D1290202

bindi

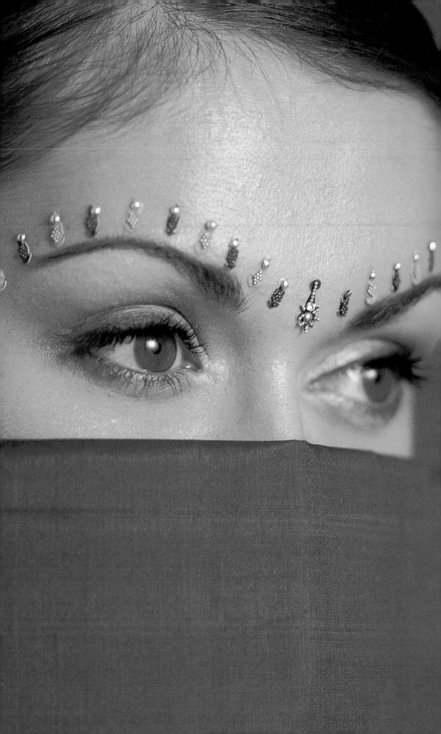

bindi

CREATE OVER
30 BODY-JEWEL DESIGNS

Beth Margetts

Journey Editions
Boston • Tokyo • Singapore

BETH MARGETTS is a freelance makeup artist and hair stylist, working in fashion, music, and at beauty exhibitions. Beth is also a trained mehndi artist.

First published in the United States in 1999 by Journey Editions, an imprint of Periplus Editions (HK) Ltd., with editorial offices at 153 Milk Street, Boston, Massachusetts 02109.

Text, design and special photography copyright © 1999 Carlton Books Limited

All rights reserved. No part of this publication may be reproduced or utilized in any form or by any means, electronic or mechanical, including photocopying, recording, or by any information storage and retrieval system, without prior written permission from Journey Editions.

Library of Congress Catalog Card Number: 99-62788

ISBN: 1-885203-98-5

Senior Executive Editor: Venetia Penfold
Art Director: Penny Stock
Editor: Lisa Dyer
Designer: Barbara Zuñiga

Picture Researcher: Alex Pepper
Production: Garry Lewis
Special Photography: Catherine Rowlands

DISTRIBUTED BY
USA
Tuttle Publishing
Distribution Center
Airport Industrial Park
364 Innovation Drive
North Clarendon, VT 05759-9436
Tel: (802) 773-8930
Tel: (800) 526-2778

Canada
Raincoast Books
8680 Cambie Street
Vancouver, British Columbia
V6P 6M9
Tel: (604) 323-7100
Fax: (604) 323-2600

Asia
Berkeley Books Pte Ltd
5 Little Road #08-01
Singapore 536983
Tel: (65) 280-3320
Fax: (65) 280-6290

The body paints and adhesives in this pack are for external use only. Take care in handling them and avoid any contact with the eyes; if you do get any of these products in your eye, wash it out immediately with cold water and, if symptoms persist, consult your doctor. As with all new skin products, do a patch test to rule out any allergic reaction. Neither the author nor the publisher is responsible for any adverse effects or consequences resulting from the use of the products in this pack.

First edition
05 04 03 02 01 00 99   10 9 8 7 6 5 4 3 2 1

Printed and bound in Italy.

Contents

Introduction 6

History 8

The western world 10

Getting started 14

Traditional and

 individual bindis 22

 traditional teardrop 22

 dressed-up drama 24

 butterfly bindi 26

 dharma dot 27

 stone bead 27

 arrow allure 28

 club chic 30

 nosestud bindi 32

 dot the eye 33

 nail magic 34

Bindi build-ups 36

 colour cross 36

 optic ornament 38

 black & white bindi 38

wedding bindi 40

purple power 42

scarlet insignia 42

a glance at glamour 44

red star 44

Diamanté bindis 46

 blue dazzle 46

 diamanté liner 48

 natural shine 50

 shimmery cheeks 51

 glitter lashes 52

 sapphire sunrise 54

 red light green light 55

Bindis and body paints 56

 bellybutton blaze 56

 navel body art 56

 tendril necklace 58

 kumkum kraze 59

 light fantastic 60

 bridal headdress 62

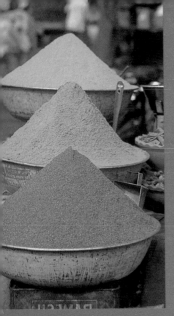

Introduction

Hot off the catwalk, bindis are the latest fashion statement to take both the stars and the starstruck by storm. Everyone is picking up on the East-meets-West theme, using ethnic ideas in clothing and accessories. Sported by actresses, television personalities, rock stars and supermodels, the bindi is a versatile body adornment that can be worn for almost any look, whether you want a traditional Indian dot for urban style or a glittery disco design for clubbing.

In this book you will find all the information you need to create a wealth of different looks using self-adhesive bindis, glue-on jewels, and body paints and powders. An opening chapter, getting started, offers you practical advice on the materials available and how to use them, along with motif ideas to help stimulate your imagination.

The designs themselves are divided into four sections. A chapter on traditional and individual bindis uses single bindis to create wildly different effects. Bindi build-ups explains how to build from simple to more complex designs using a pack of self-adhesive bindis. Diamanté bindis shows how to

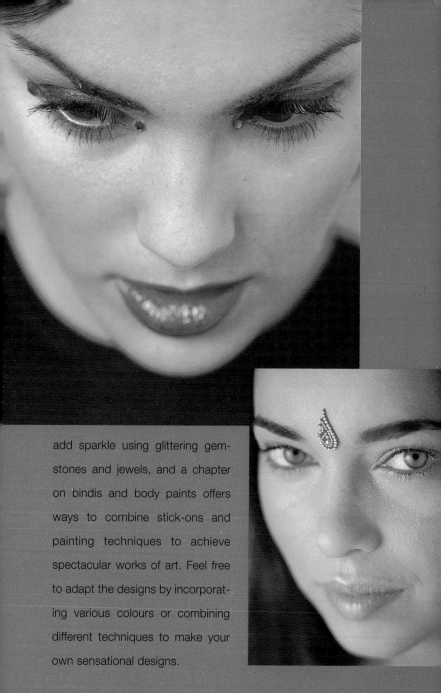

add sparkle using glittering gemstones and jewels, and a chapter
on bindis and body paints offers
ways to combine stick-ons and
painting techniques to achieve
spectacular works of art. Feel free
to adapt the designs by incorporat-
ing various colours or combining
different techniques to make your
own sensational designs.

History

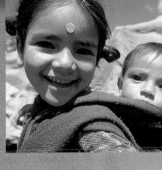

Wearing a jewel in the centre of the forehead originates from the red dot worn by married women in India. As part of the Hindu marriage ceremony, a dot of red kumkum, a powder made from flower petals, was pressed into the forehead. Gradually other colours of kumkum

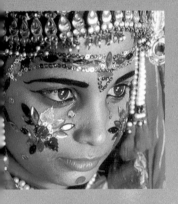

powder were developed and Indian women could match their bindi to the outfit they were wearing. As time went on and Indian dress became more elaborate, body jewels in various colours and designs were produced. Today, self-adhesive bindis are an important part of the Indian woman's dress, but they have also become popular with the fashion-conscious.

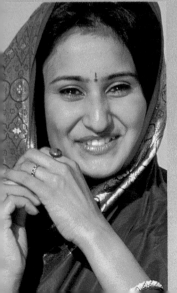

Traditionally a Hindu bride wears an ornate arrangement of bindis that curves over the eyebrows and sweeps across the forehead. Known as the 'wedding bindi', this design has been copied by young trendsetters, though a simple solo bindi remains the most wearable style.

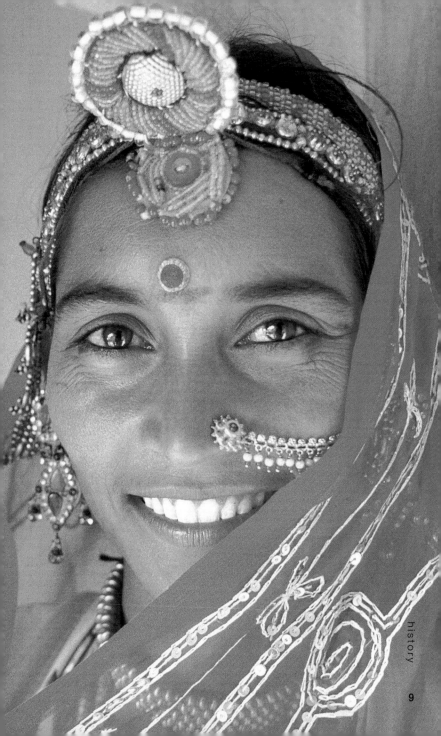

The Western World

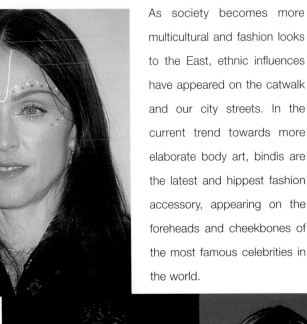

As society becomes more multicultural and fashion looks to the East, ethnic influences have appeared on the catwalk and our city streets. In the current trend towards more elaborate body art, bindis are the latest and hippest fashion accessory, appearing on the foreheads and cheekbones of the most famous celebrities in the world.

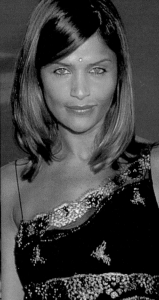

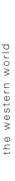

10

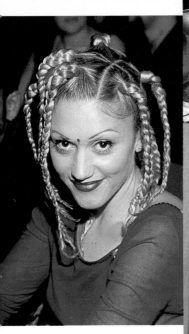

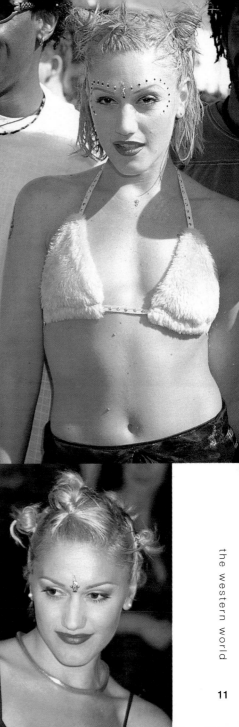

Opposite top With two decades in the limelight, Madonna opts yet again to ride the waves of fashion.

Opposite bottom Helena Christensen coordinates slinky saris and beaded dresses with bindi accessories.

This page Gwen Stefani works bindis into her diverse wardrobes.

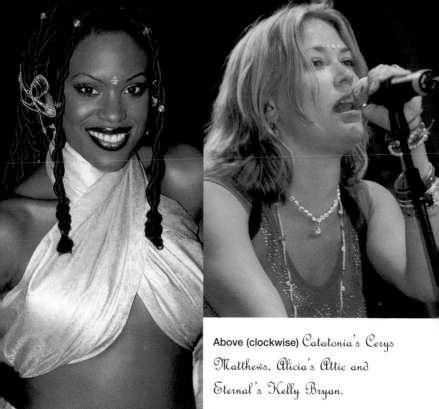

Above (clockwise) Catatonia's Cerys Matthews, Alicia's Attic and Eternal's Kelly Bryan.

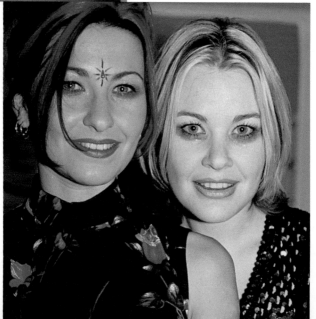

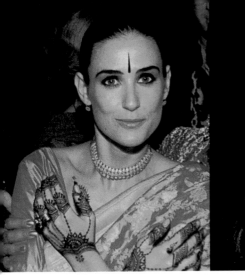

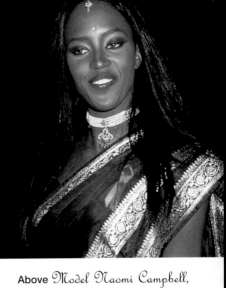

Above Reflecting a very 1990s theme of East-meets-West, Demi Moore shows off a star's style.
Below Always uniting the spiritual with the stylish, Boy George sports some simple bindis.

Above Model Naomi Campbell, lover of all things Eastern, wears a traditional bindi.
Below Model Sophie Dahl matches bindi to necklace to show that black is always in vogue.

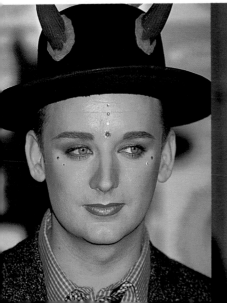

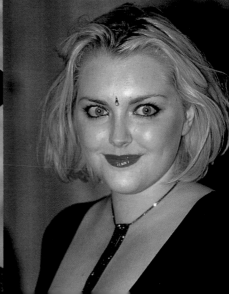

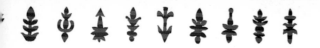

getting started

Bindis are a fun, easy way to transform your look and a great way to spice up a style for a party. Whether you decide to reproduce an ornate design or just want a few little diamantés to decorate your cheek, all you need are some basic materials and a little patience.

bindis

Self-adhesive bindis are available in packs from department stores, pharmacies, accessory shops, or specialist Indian or sari shops. All shapes and sizes can be found, from tiny pearls to large teardrops and crosses to more specific shapes such as butterflies, flowers, crescent moons or stars. Any gemstone, as long as it is flat-backed, can be used for a bindi. Diamantés in particular are a popular choice, since their colour and size range is wide; they can be obtained either

  individually or in packs from jewellery and costume suppliers. You can find bindis that are flat, faceted or beaded, or ones that are holograms, gemstones or crystal. Special navel bindis, flat and large enough to cover the belly-button, are also available, as are stick-on nail bindis which bend to the contours of the nail. (See page 64 for information on sourcing bindis.)

tips

• Match makeup and clothing to the bindi, but keep a balanced look. Dark-coloured bindis need dramatic makeup. Glittery jewels need shimmer and shine.

• Choose a bindi that complements your overall look and personality, whether hippie chic, glamour puss, minimalist, party girl or urban street.

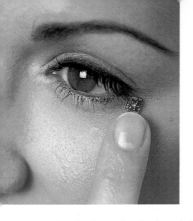

applying bindis

The easiest bindis to use are self-adhesive, but many others, such as gemstones and diamantés, can be applied with false-eyelash or latex glue. All bindis should be added after makeup is completed. Bindis are not just for decorating the face, but can form designs on the wrist, ankle, neck or shoulder – anywhere you want a little decoration, just make sure the area is free of clothing.

• Peel a self-adhesive bindi from the pack and stick it on clean, dry skin with a fingertip (above) – the bindi may fall off recently moisturized skin. Tweezers are useful for positioning very tiny stick-ons.

• For flat-backed gemstones, pick up the bindi with tweezers, dab on a little false-eyelash or latex glue, then press into position (below). The bindi can be removed with makeup remover or a daily cleanser.

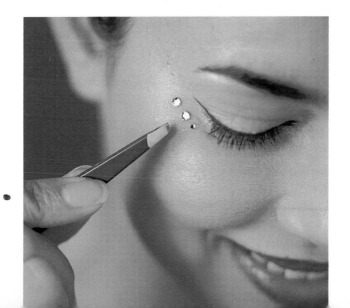

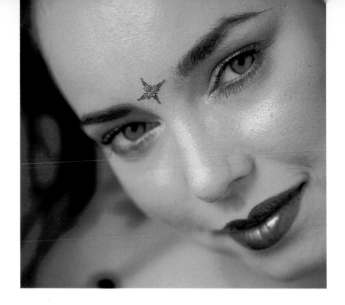

building up bindis

Many self-adhesive bindis are sold in packs for the traditional wedding bindi. These include a large ornate jewel for the centre of the design and 20 or more smaller jewels. The packs can be broken down or built up to create endless variations. You may like to use just the large bindi in a central position between the brows, then build up your own design around it using two or more of the smaller ones. Move the bindis to different positions until you get the composition you want.

Bindi designs look best with the thickest part of the jewel facing towards the centre of the face or the design, with smaller, narrower jewels tapering away or radiating out from the middle. Teardrop or oblong shapes look great when positioned next to rounded shapes or flower bindis.

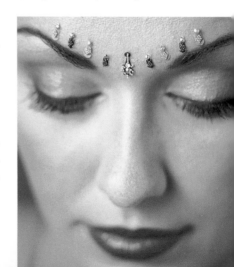

body paints

Kumkum powder or bindi paints in various colours are the most traditional method of painting on bindis, but you may want to experiment with glitter, ultraviolet paints, henna or any of the special body-art pens available from pharmacies. Eye pencils or liquid eyeliners also work extremely well. Avoid greasepaint, though, as it is more apt to smear and much harder to remove than other body paints. When using any form of body paint, do a patch test first to check for an allergic reaction. Do this by applying a small amount of paint to the skin and waiting for 24 hours; if any redness develops, do not use the paint. Work on clean, dry skin and lightly sketch out your design with an eyebrow pencil if you feel unsure about working freehand. After completing the design, allow your work to dry thoroughly, and take care to close up the paints tightly so they do not dry out.

using stencils

Stencils offer a foolproof method of painting on a bindi that is ideal for the beginner or those unsure of drawing designs freehand. Metal or card stencils are usually included with liquid or powder body paints, but you can make your own by tracing a design onto cardboard and then cutting out specific areas. For best results, remember to organize your paints or powders first so they are close at hand. The stencil should be held firmly against the skin with one hand while you brush on the colour with your other hand. Use a fine-tipped artist's paintbrush and make sure that all the areas to be coloured are completely filled in before lifting off the stencil, taking care not to smudge the design.

getting started

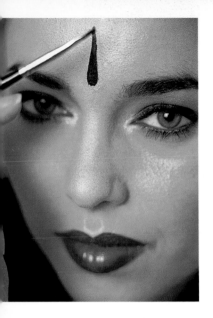

bindi paints

Specialist liquid bindi paints are based on the traditional kumkum powder and are available in a range of colours from pharmacies and accessory shops. Any water-soluble body paints can be substituted. The paint can be removed with soap and water or your daily cleanser. Using bindi paints in combination with stick-ons offers endless creative possibilities.

kumkum powder

Available as fine loose powder, kumkum is best used with a stencil to create a soft, subtle, broken effect. Because it is the authentic bindi powder, it will fall off slightly during application. Petroleum jelly needs to be dabbed on first to hold the colour and you will need to brush on quite a lot of powder before removing the stencil. To catch any surplus colour that may fall onto the under-eye area, brush it with talcum powder first. The colour will fall onto the talcum, which can then be easily brushed away.

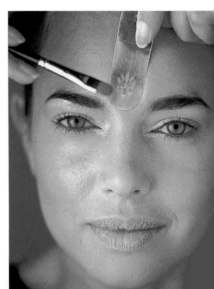

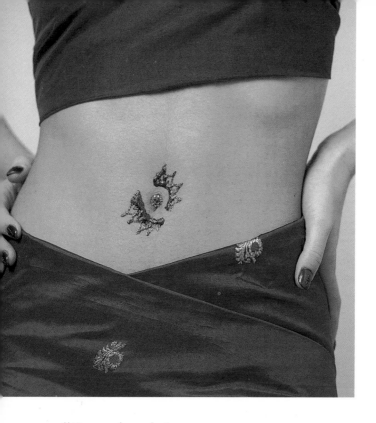

glittered paints

The trend for all things that shimmer and glitter in cosmetics is evident in body paints too. Vibrant glitter colours are perfect for creating a party look. Use glitter paints as you would the bindi paints, but remember that a little goes a long way. Avoid using too many different colours in one design or combining the paint with too much glittery makeup. A good idea is to embellish a design painted in matt colours with a little glitter here and there. The glittered paints are water-soluble and can be removed with soap and water or a daily cleanser, though the glitter particles themselves have a tendency to cling to the skin.

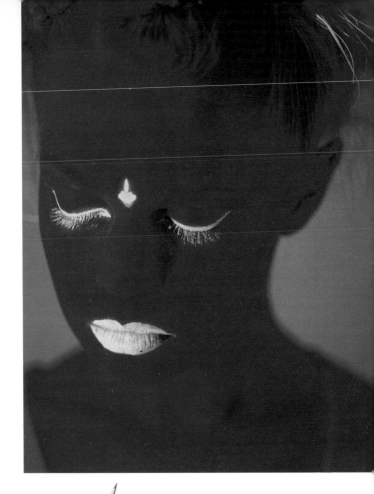

uv paints

For a fun night out, experiment with the ultra-violet body paints available to create painted bindis or body art. The best ones to use are those that show up as a colour when you apply them, but glow under the ultraviolet light in clubs. The clear version is much more difficult to use accurately and you will have to wait until you are under UV lights to see the fruits of your labour.

painting bindis

Use bindi paints or powder, ultraviolet or glitter paints, or just a simple eyeliner in your favourite colour to recreate the designs featured here. Some of the motifs may give you inspiration for more involved body art designs, or work several ideas together. Many of the designs in the next chapter can be painted on instead of stuck on. Alternatively, you may like to draw designs such as swirls, bullseyes or semi-circles around self-adhesive bindis, or draw arrows or lines through them.

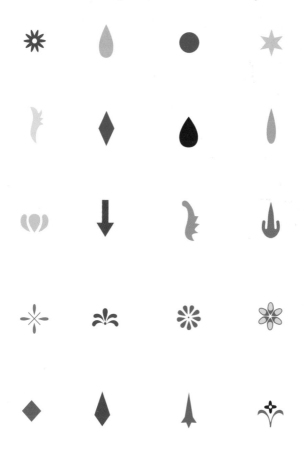

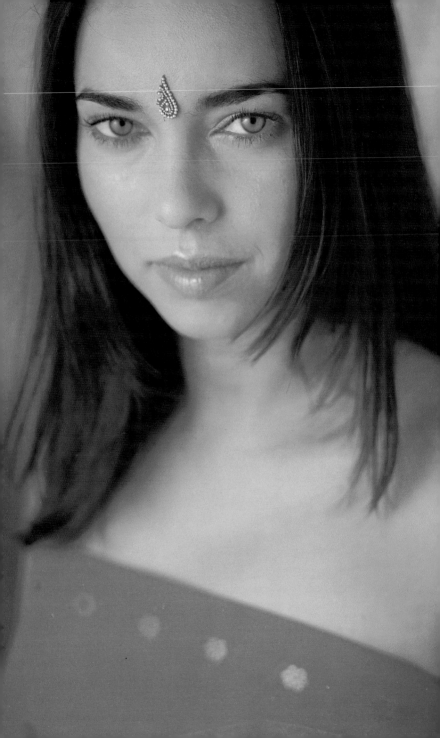

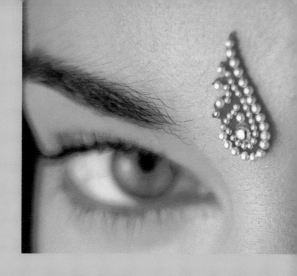

traditional teardrop

This red and pearl bindi is best worn solo to show off its classic teardrop shape and ornate detail.

Get the look

◊ Stick the self-adhesive bindi in position, centred between the eyebrows. Because it is very large, the bindi needs to be placed slightly low down, towards the nose.

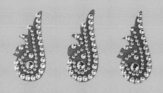

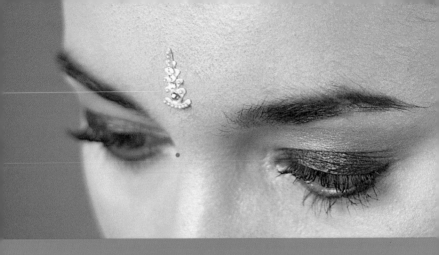

dressed-up drama

A clear crystal bindi in an anchor shape is elegant on its own and the perfect adornment for a special evening out.

Get the look

- ◊ Stick the self-adhesive bindi in position, centred between the eyebrows but slightly above the browline. Make sure the narrowest part of the bindi points towards the hairline.

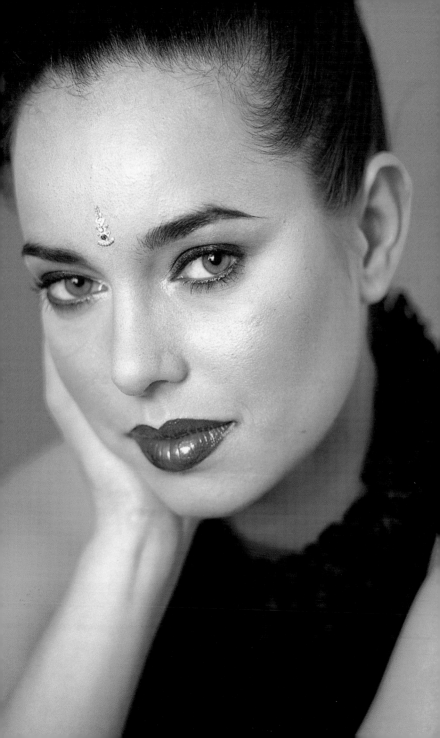

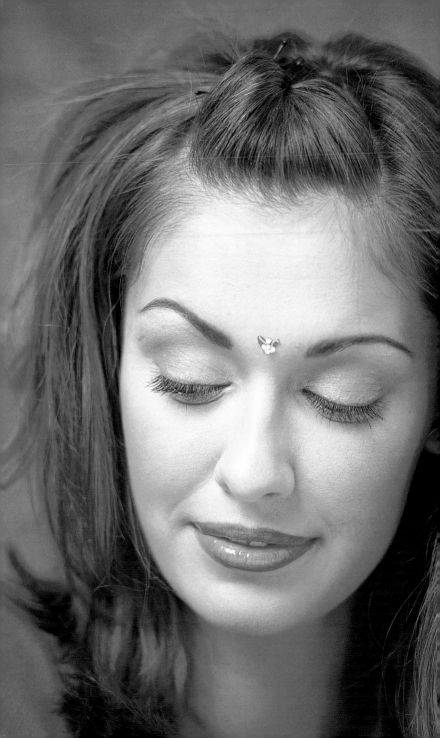

butterfly bindi

Motifs such as butterflies, hearts and stars are available as stick-on bindis and can be placed anywhere on the body. Here a butterfly creates a fun, fresh look.

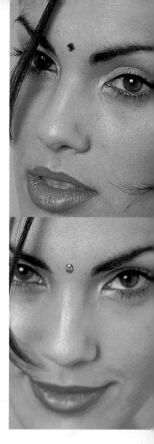

dharma dot

A simple brown gemstone bindi, combined with natural makeup and healthy glowing skin, creates a beautiful pure effect that would be ideal for the daytime.

stone bead

For an urban look that is down to earth but slightly glamorous, choose a silvery bead bindi. Use pretty pastel makeup and silver jewellery to finish off.

Get the look

◊ For all the designs featured here, stick the self-adhesive bindi in position, centred between the eyebrows.

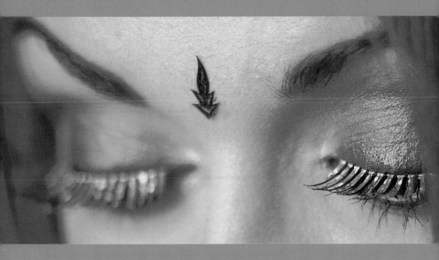

arrow allure

Create a glamorous gothic look by choosing a dark-coloured bindi that is complemented by dramatic makeup and false lashes.

Get the look

◊ Stick the self-adhesive bindi in position, centred between the eyebrows with the arrow pointing towards the nose.

◊ Complete the effect by adding false glitter lashes and using deep plum colours for eyes and lips.

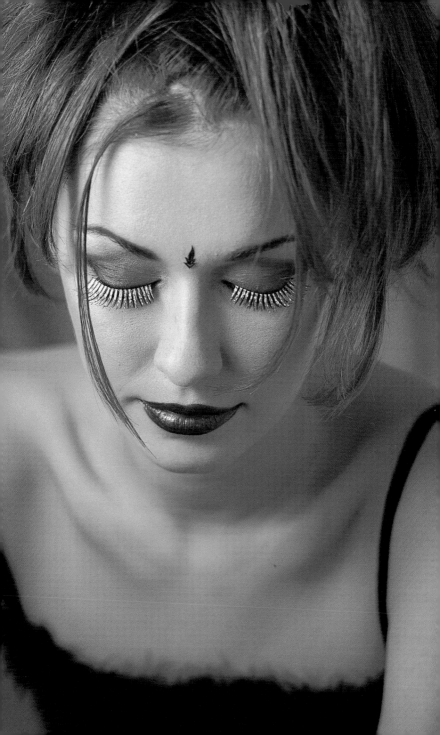

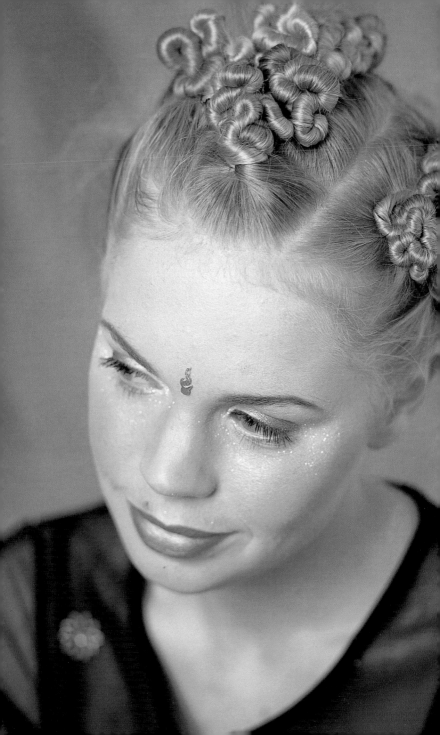

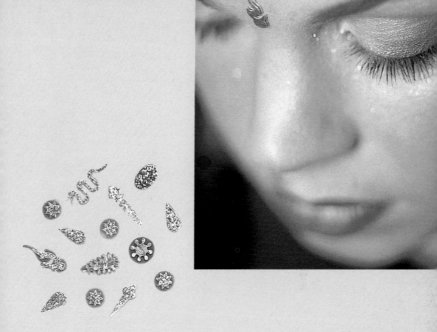

club chic

This clubby look is created by using a swirly silvery bindi combined with makeup in pale iridescent colours. If you like, add smaller silver bindis in different shapes to cheekbones and brush on some glitter dust to sparkle the night away.

Get the look

� Stick the self-adhesive silver bindi in position, centrally between the eyebrows and with the narrow end pointing towards the hairline.

traditional and individual bindis

31

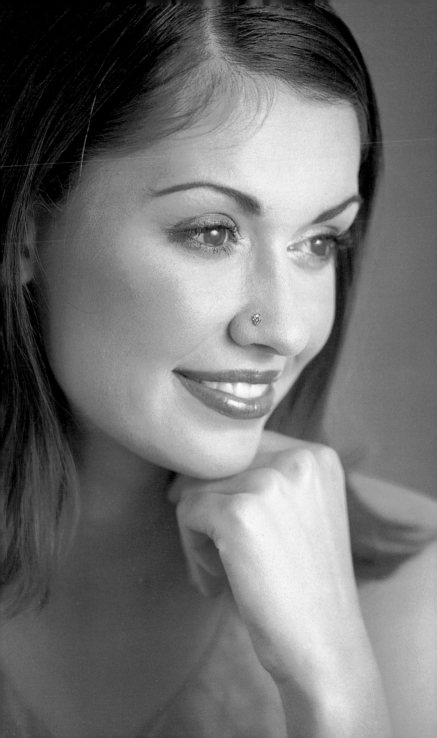

nosestud bindi

Using a bindi is a great way to experiment with a nosestud without the permanence of piercing.

Get the look

- Choose a tiny self-adhesive bindi and stick in position on the side of the nose.

dot the eye

A jewel placed near the eye is a subtle way of drawing other people's attention to you.

Get the look

- Stick a square-cut self-adhesive bindi in position on the lower outer corner of the eye.

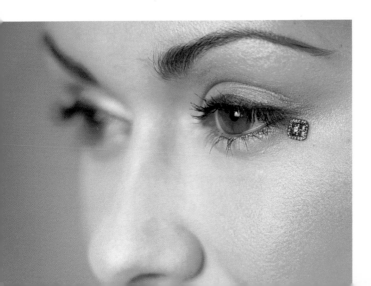

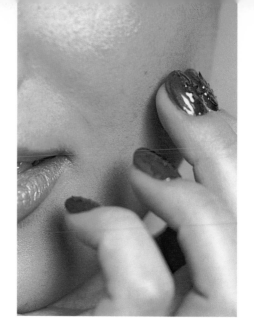

nail magic

This design uses self-adhesive bindis made specifically for the nails, which are flat but will bend to the contours of the nail. Try using different combinations of nail colours and bindis on each finger for a more funky feel.

Get the look

- ◊ Paint a dark scarlet nail polish on all your nails. Allow to dry.

- ◊ Carefully apply a bindi to each nail, making sure the stick-on is straight and smooth.

- ◊ Seal your nails with a coat of clear nail polish and allow to dry.

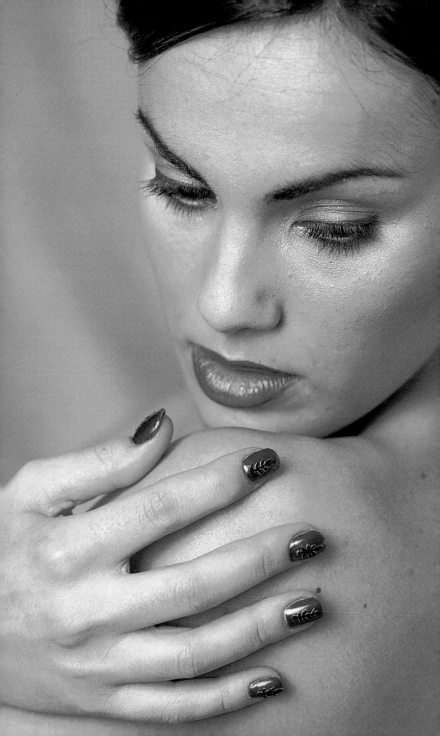

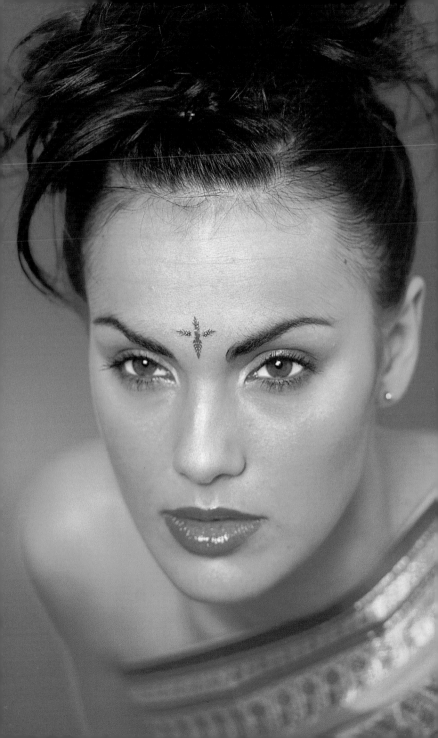

colour cross

Only four small bindis from a full pack are used here, and the dot is painted on. You may find it helpful to place the bottom section of the cross first before adding the dot and the remaining bindis.

Get the look

- Using body paints, paint a red dot centrally between the eyebrows, above the browline.

- Using the red dot as the centre, stick on a green self-adhesive bindi vertically below the red dot. Add the three remaining bindis to make a cross formation.

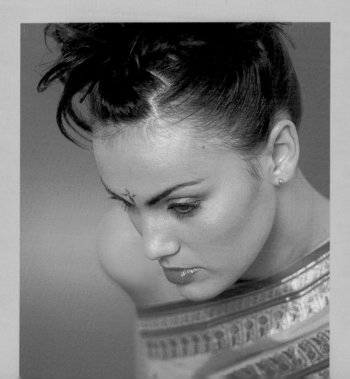

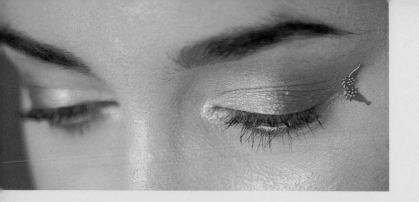

optic ornament

Two bindis form an arrow pointing directly towards the eye. What better way to get someone special to look at you?

Get the look
- Stick two small red self-adhesive bindis at right angles to each other on the outer corner of the eye, making sure the narrowest part of the bindis are facing away from the eye.

black & white bindi

Here a pretty pearl bindi is extended and 'framed' by adding two smaller black bindis.

Get the look
- Stick on the large self-adhesive bindi, centred between the eyebrows and slightly above the browline. Then place the two smaller bindis above and below to create a linear effect.

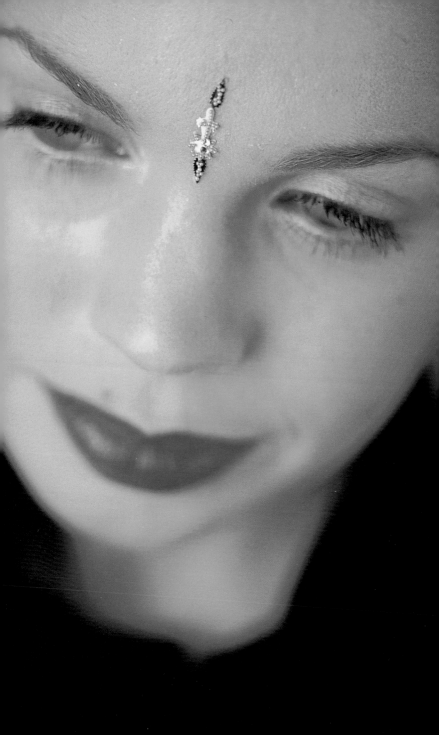

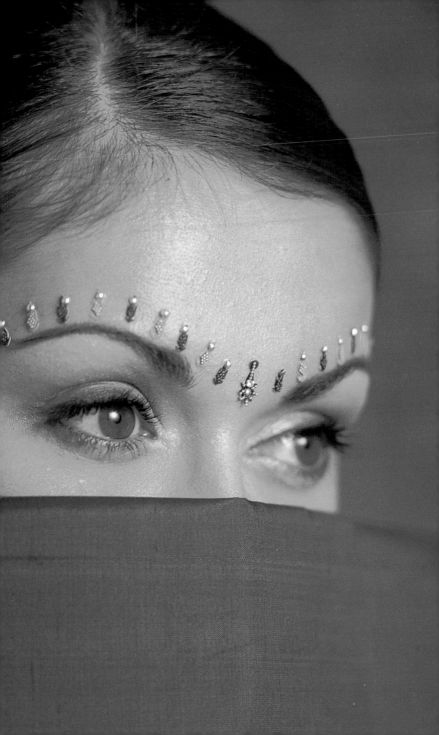

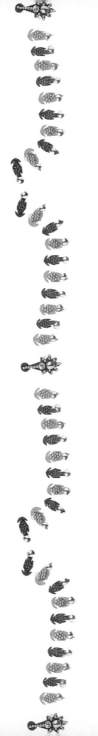

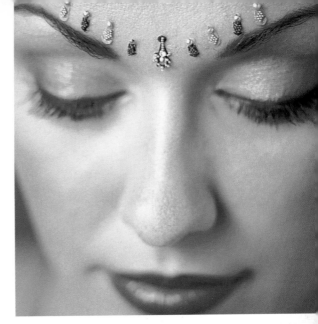

wedding bindi

A more simplified and wearable version of the traditional wedding bindi, this design uses the full wedding pack of 21 stick-ons.

Get the look

- ❀ Stick the large bindi in position, centrally between the eyebrows.

- ❀ Add the smaller bindis in alternating colours, working in both directions from the centre out and following the arch of the brows.

- ❀ For a less complicated look, stop the line one-third or halfway across the browline.

bindi build-ups

41

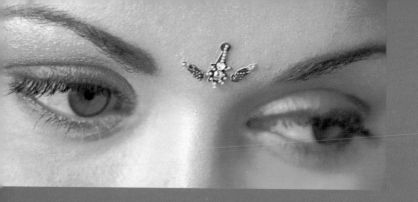

purple power

An arrow shape follows the natural lines of the brows and is one of the most popular bindi designs.

Get the look

◊ Stick a large black and gold self-adhesive bindi in position, centrally between the eyebrows.

◊ Add two purple bindis left and right of the base of the central bindi and pointing out at angles to form an arrow formation.

 # **scarlet** insignia

For this design, the central bindi must have two beads to achieve a balanced effect.

Get the look

◊ Stick a large red double-beaded self-adhesive bindi in position, centrally between the eyebrows. Add two smaller red bindis left and right of the central bindi but above the lowest bead.

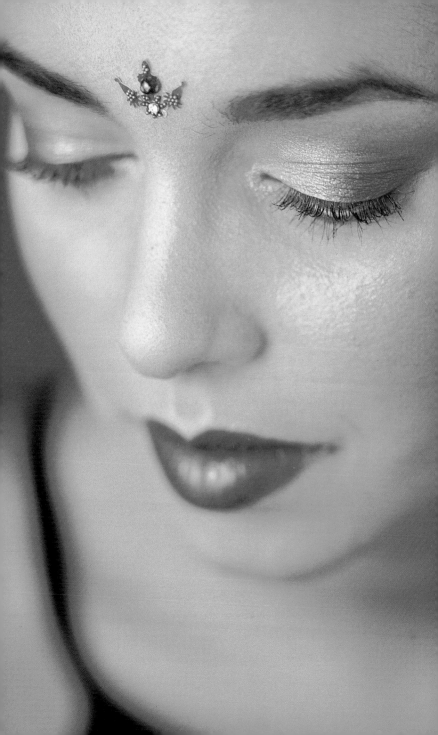

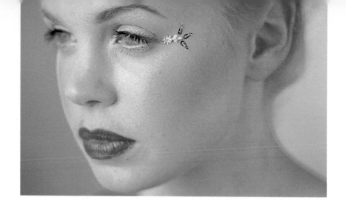

a glance at glamour

For ornate bindi designs, make sure you treat both eyes exactly the same or the result will look lopsided.

Get the look

- Stick the large self-adhesive bindi at the outer corner of the eye with the cross section pointing towards the hairline. Add three small bindis to radiate out from the large bindi.

red star

Four bindis create a star with a beaded centre that looks stunning day or night.

Get the look

- Stick one red self-adhesive bindi in position, centrally between the eyebrows with the thickest end pointing towards the hairline.
- Add three more bindis to create a cross, overlapping the ends to fill in the centre of the design.

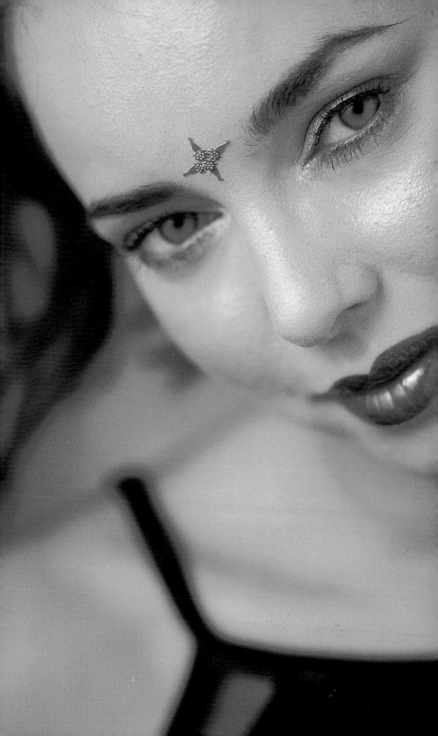

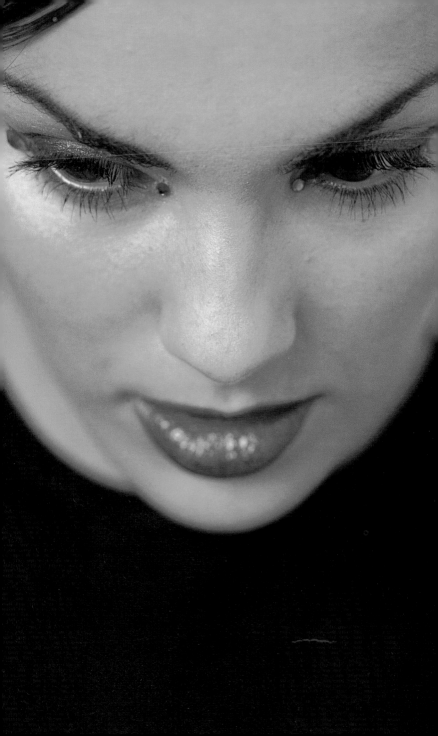

blue dazzle

Take care to position the bindis correctly. If they are too low, the eyes will look droopy. You will need two small and two large blue diamanté jewels.

Get the look

◊ With an eyebrow pencil, lightly mark the desired positions for the bindis in the inner and outer corners of the eyes.

◊ Place a dab of eyelash glue on the back of a small jewel, then press it onto the inner corner of the eye. Apply glue to the large jewel and position it on the outer corner of the eye. Repeat for the other eye.

◊ Complete the look by sweeping electric blue eyeliner across the top eyelids.

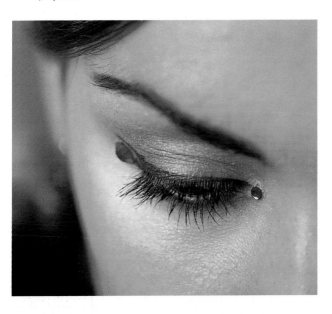

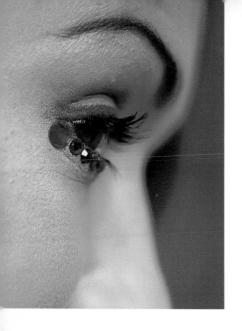

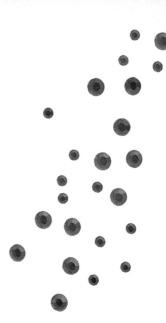

diamanté liner

A row of red diamantés creates a sparkling line under the eye. Only small and medium-size jewels were used in this design, but you could incorporate three or four different sizes.

Get the look

- ◊ With an eyebrow pencil, lightly mark the desired positions for the diamantés, making sure they are evenly spaced and the same on both eyes.

- ◊ Place a dab of eyelash glue on the back of a small jewel. Press into the position closest to the nose. Add small jewels in a row, working outwards, then finish with a large diamanté at the outer corner of the eye. Repeat for the other eye.

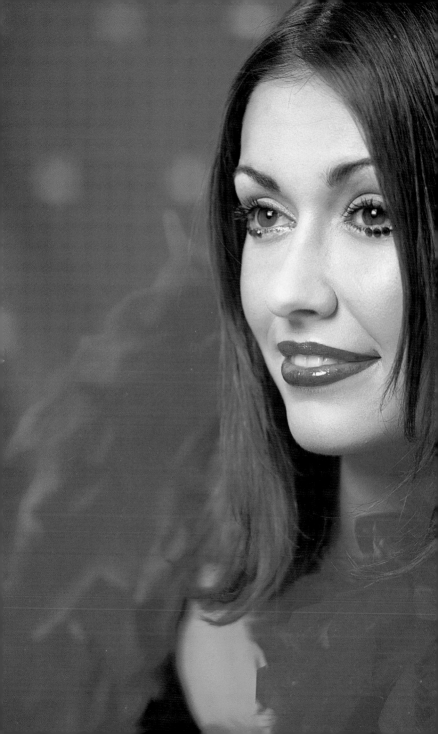

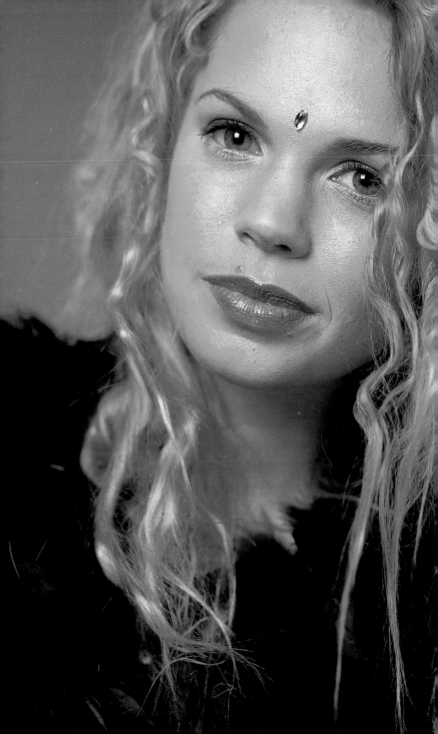

shimmery
cheeks

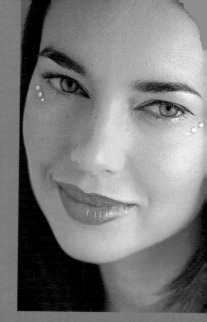

Enhance your dazzling good looks with an idea taken straight from the catwalk.

Get the look

- With an eyebrow pencil, lightly mark three positions for the bindis on the area between the eye and the cheek-bone on each side of the face.

- Place a dab of eyelash glue on the back of a small jewel. Press into the position furthest from the eye. Add a medium-sized jewel in the next position and finish with the largest jewel closest to the eye. Repeat for the other cheek.

natural shine

A simple sparkling diamanté in an oval shape adds a special touch to a subtle look, especially when combined with light-reflecting makeup.

Get the look

- With an eyebrow pencil, mark a position for the bindi centrally between eyebrows. Place a dab of eyelash glue on the back of a clear silvery diamanté gemstone and press in place.

diamanté bindis

51

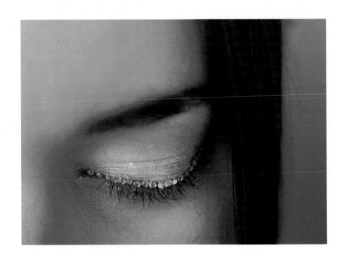

glitter lashes

Very tiny diamantés are used here, fitted tightly together next to the lashes, to create a disco diva design. You will need 20-30 jewels per eye and a fair amount of patience.

Get the look

- ◊ Place a little eyelash glue on the back of your left hand. Pick up a tiny diamanté with tweezers, dab the back carefully in the glue, then press into the inner corner of the eye as close to the lashes as possible.

- ◊ Continue adding jewels one at a time, working from the inner eye outwards and making sure there are no gaps between the diamantés. Repeat for the other eye.

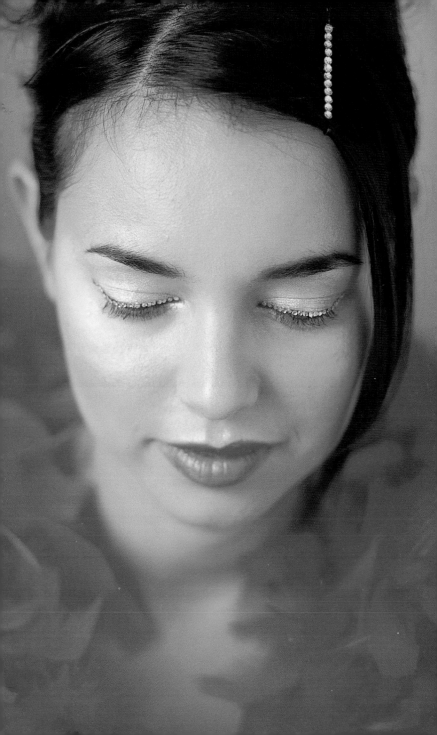

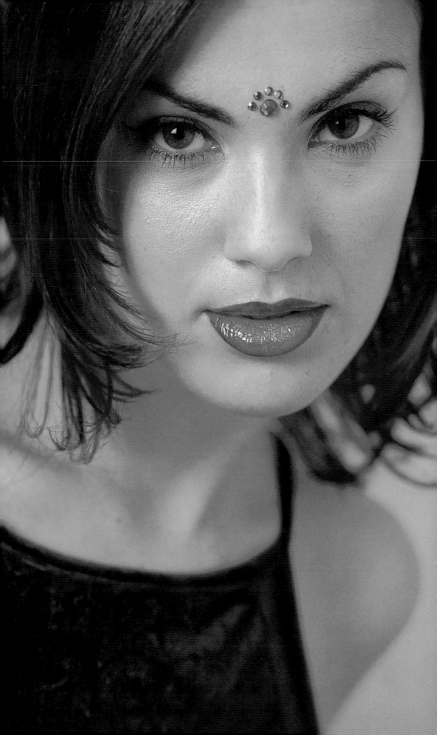

red light
green light

Glittering diamanté bindis glow traffic-light red and green.

Get the look

❧ Using slightly tacky eyelash glue, place a dab of glue on the back of a red jewel. Press it into position just to the left of the centre point between the eyebrows. Add another red jewel above the first.

❧ Repeat for the green jewels, working to the right of the centre and adding three diamantés to the tier.

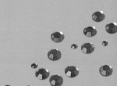

sapphire sunrise

This design gives the impression of the sun rising over the horizon, but for a different effect place the smaller diamantés in a cross formation around the central bindi.

Get the look

❧ With an eyebrow pencil, lightly mark the central position for the large bindi. Place a dab of eyelash glue on the back of the large diamanté bindi and press it in place.

❧ Glue four small round diamantés in a semi-circle around the top of the central bindi.

diamanté bindis

bellybutton blaze

Light up under the nightclub rays by using a special UV navel bindi in combination with UV body paints and nail polish.

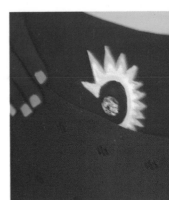

Get the look

- Stick a self-adhesive UV bindi on the navel, making sure it is large enough to cover it.
- Using UV body paints in yellows and reds, paint a swirl around the navel, then build up the design with spikes in different colours.

navel body art

Any design that draws attention to the navel bindi works well. You may like to try a complete circle or paint a line or arrow going through the navel.

Get the look

- Stick a self-adhesive blue jewel bindi on the navel, making sure it is large enough to cover it completely.
- Using glitter body paints in purple and green, paint two semi-circles around the navel, leaving a gap between them. Add pointed leaf shapes radiating outwards.

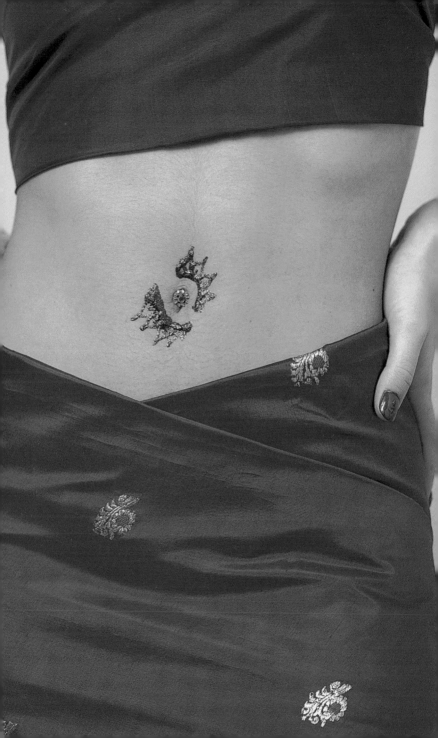

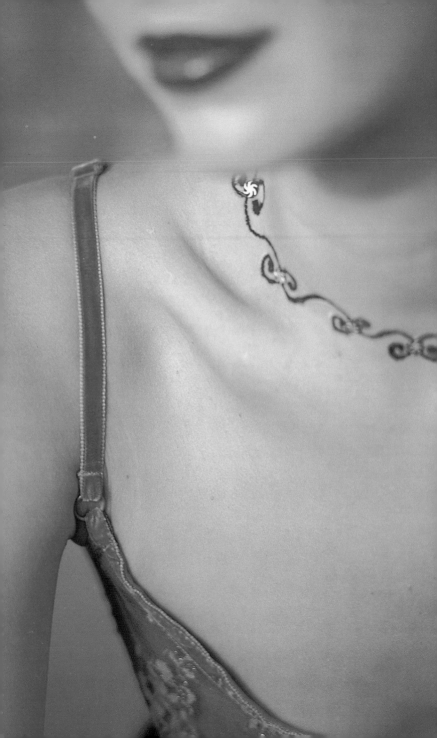

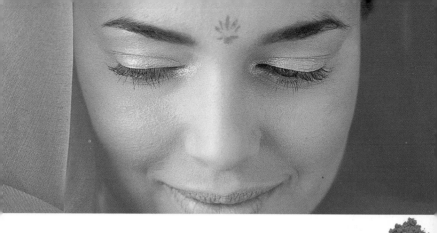

kumkum kraze

You can use one colour of kumkum, overlayer a few, or fill in sections of the stencil in different colours.

Get the look

❦ Dab a thin layer of petroleum jelly over the design area. Holding the stencil in position, apply yellow powder, then layer orange powder on top (see pages 17-18). Carefully remove the stencil.

tendril necklace

Here a delicate painted necklace is enhanced with stick-on bindis. You may need the help of a friend!

Get the look

❦ Using an eyebrow pencil, draw connecting swirls around the neck. Paint the design using a fine brush and purple body paints. When dry, stick self-adhesive bindis at the points where the swirls meet.

bindis and body paints

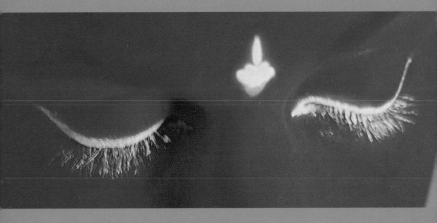

light fantastic

Make an impact on the dance floor with this artful bindi, created with an arrow stencil and UV body paints in a trio of colours.

Get the look

- ⬥ With one hand, firmly hold a stencil in position on your forehead. Using a fine brush, fill in areas of the stencil with red, green and orange ultraviolet body paint.
- ⬥ Carefully remove the stencil.
- ⬥ To complete the overall effect, use ultraviolet makeup to line your eyes and colour in your lashes and lips.

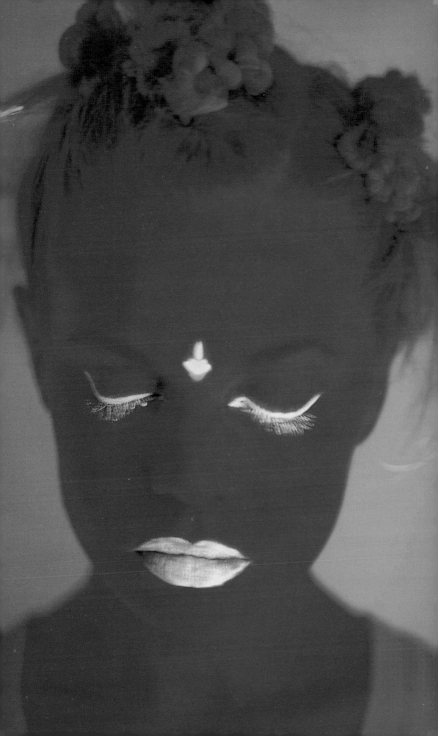

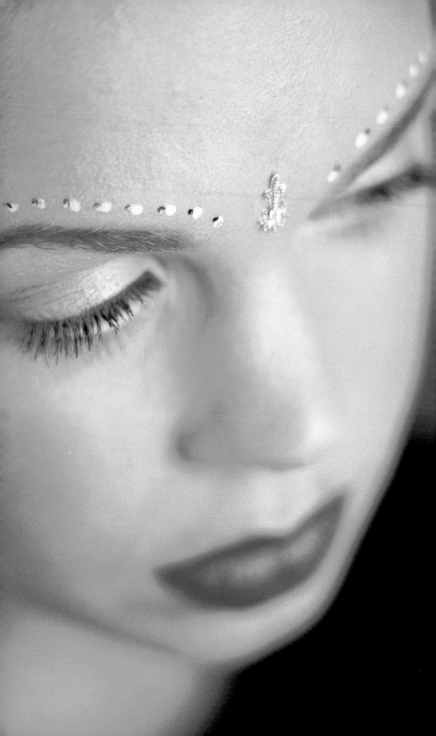

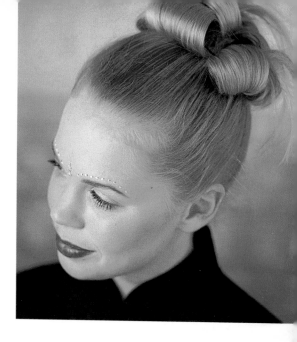

bridal headdress

This traditional design combines a stick-on bindi with body paints, but you may like to alternate dots of paint with stick-on jewels or paint on dots in different colours.

Get the look

- ❀ With an eyebrow pencil, lightly mark the positions for the design. Stick a white and gold self-adhesive bindi in position, centrally between the eyebrows.

- ❀ Using white body paint, paint on large white dots over each eyebrow, working in both directions from the centre out and following the arch of the brows. When dry, paint on tiny black dots in the corner of each white one.